Frenc
Cuisi

GU01017805

Contents

Intention of this Guide

This guide—*French and Italian Cuisine Passport,* is intended to provide information useful to people living with food allergies and specialized diets. AllergyFree Passport™, LLC as the authors, R & R Publishing, LLC as the publisher, the contributors and reviewers of this guide (collectively "we") have made reasonable efforts to make sure that the information provided is accurate and complete. We believe that factual information contained in this guide was correct to the best of our knowledge at the time of publication. However, we do not warrant or guarantee that any of the information is accurate or complete. It is not possible for us to have gathered all the information available or independently analyzed or tested the information.

We assume no responsibility for errors, inaccuracies, omissions or typographical errors contained in this guide. We expressly disclaim responsibility for any adverse effects arising from the use or application of the information contained herein, as well as responsibility for any liability, injury, loss or damage, whether it be actual, special, consequential, personal or otherwise, which is incurred or allegedly incurred as a direct or indirect consequence of the use and application of any of the contents of this guide or for references made within it.

The information contained in this guide should not be viewed as medical advice. Questions regarding specific food allergies, specialized diets, drug and food interactions and anything related to a specific individual should be addressed to a doctor or other medical practitioner.

We are not responsible for any goods and/or services referred to in this guide. By providing this information, we do not endorse any business or advocate the use of any products or services referred to in this guide, and the owners or operators of the businesses referred to in this guide do not endorse AllergyFree Passport™, LLC or R & R Publishing, LLC. We expressly disclaim any liability relating to the use of any goods and/or services referred to in this guide.

Although the authors and the publishers of this guide are appreciative of the support and information received, AllergyFree Passport™, LLC and R & R Publishing, LLC are not affiliated with (and have not received any compensation from or related to) any of the individuals, restaurants or businesses identified in this guide.

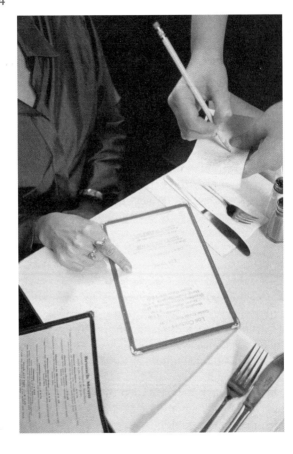

"If I have helped just one person in exploring a new location, be it in the city or country side, within their own country and/or on foreign lands, I will feel as though I have succeeded."
—Ralph Waldo Emerson

Passport Introduction

Overview

As part of the *Let's Eat Out!* Series, the *French and Italian Cuisine Passport* is the first pocket reference guide dedicated to eating outside the home by respective cuisine while managing 10 common food allergens including: corn, dairy, eggs, fish, gluten, peanuts, shellfish, soy, tree nuts and wheat. This pioneering effort focuses on what you can eat by providing allergy considerations for 60-plus sample menu items from these two international cuisines. The contents of this passport are based on years of personal experience, extensive research, proven results and the collaborative efforts of many individuals and organizations around the world. This light-weight passport is designed to facilitate a safe eating experience whether you are traveling around the corner from your home or around the world.

Passport Approach

The passport is organized in a manner that allows you to use the information in a number of different ways. One of our key guiding principles was to develop an easy-to-use guide that is succinct and flexible to meet an individual's needs. It can be read cover to cover as a reference guide or if you prefer, you can skip around depending upon what cuisine or menu items you are most interested in learning about. For example, if you're planning to go to a restaurant, you may want to learn about the cuisine, potential menu items, associated guidelines and how to navigate through the restaurant menu. If you just need to re-familiarize yourself on possible choices or want a "cheat sheet" to bring with you to help guide your choices, you can view the *Quick Reference Guides*. It's all about your needs, preferences and areas of concern during that particular moment of the day.

Design and Methodology

The format is standardized across the cuisines, allowing you, the reader to easily recognize each section of information. The *Dining Considerations* outline how menus may be presented as well as relevant cultural customs and service styles for each cuisine. The *Sample Cuisine Menus* identify the name of each dish in its native language with the English equivalent. In our global research, we discovered that international cuisines often present each menu item in the language of the country you are in, as well as the native language. We researched cuisine menus and recipes from all over the world to determine which items are most commonly found in each cuisine. Once established, we reviewed each menu item to determine which dishes had the highest likelihood of being gluten/wheat-free. We further narrowed the selection by determining which menu items had the highest likelihood of not including the eight other common food allergens discussed in this passport.

Cuisine Menu Item Descriptions summarize each dish's ingredients and the culinary preparation techniques involved in its creation. We determined what areas of food preparation had to be confirmed with the restaurant to ensure each dish was gluten/wheat-free, what other common food allergens could be potentially included and the areas of food preparation that must be questioned to ensure an allergy-free dining experience. After each description, we outline the following concerns:

Gluten-Free Decision Factors:
- "Ensure" an ingredient is not present as part of the food preparation

- "Request" an item is not included or inquire about a substitution

Food Allergen Preparation Considerations:
- "Contains" an allergen from an ingredient in alphabetical order

- "May contain" an allergen from an ingredient in alphabetical order

The *Cuisine Quick Reference Guides* are designed to give you easy access to information discussed in the menu item descriptions. It provides an overview of each item in the sample menus and indicates whether a dish "typically contains" or "may contain" an allergen. These guides highlight what you need to be aware of to order applicable menu items, avoid specific allergens and adhere to your specialized diet at a glance.

About the Authors and Additional Products outlines background details and product information.

This passport can be used as a daily resource, a reference guide, an educational tool or a training manual depending upon your perspective. We hope it meets your diverse needs and empowers you with the knowledge to achieve your desired gluten and allergy-free objectives.

And remember,

**"Life loves to be taken by
the lapel and told,
'I am with you kid. Let's go!'"**
– Maya Angelou

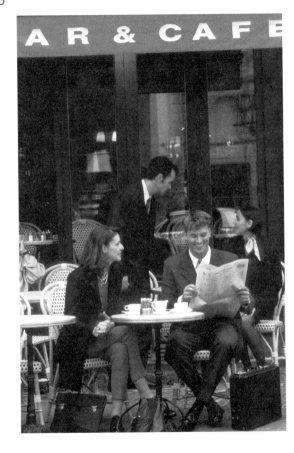

Eating is a serious venture,
if not a patriotic duty, in France.
—Patricia Roberts

Let's Eat French Cuisine

Cuisine Overview

The following materials outline:

- Dining considerations
- Sample French menu
- French cuisine menu items and descriptions
- Quick reference guide

Dining Considerations

French menu items are usually presented in the French language. You often find menu descriptions in the language of the country you are in following the name of the French menu item. While traveling, be sure to familiarize yourself with the common French culinary terms included in this chapter to assist you in your dining experience.

French restaurants serve their cuisine in a style known as *service à la russe,* which is the practice of serving a meal in many courses. Previously, the French dined in a fashion much closer to our modern buffets. Today, the standard French lunch or dinner begins with *hors d'oeuvres* and is followed by soup, main course, salad, cheese and dessert. This multi-course plan was adapted from the Russian culture during the Napoleonic wars in the 19th century and remains the standard for our modern French gastronomic experience.

The French generally eat three meals a day. *Le petit déjeuner* is a light breakfast and usually consists of bread, cereals, fruit and coffee. *Le déjeuner* takes place between noon and 2 p.m. and is a larger meal, often consisting of three courses including soup, salad and a main dish. *Le goûter* is a snack sometimes taken in the late afternoon. The French dinner or *le dîner* is preceded by *l'apéritif*, a national custom that involves setting aside half an hour or so before a meal to share a drink, small appetizers and conversation with family, friends, neighbors or colleagues. *Le dîner* is a long affair, complete with many courses and lasts two to four hours; thereby allowing ample time to enjoy and savor the meal. It is also a time for the whole family to gather together and talk about their day. Wine is enjoyed throughout the evening, with after dinner drinks such as *calvados*, *cognac* and *eaux de vie* reserved for the end of the meal.

Bon Appetit!

Sample French Menu

Appetizers

Crevette Cocktail (Shrimp Cocktail)
Escargot (Snails)
Foies Gras (Fat Liver)
Les Huîtres (Oysters on the Half Shell)
Steak Tartare (Beef Tartar)
Tartare de Saumon (Salmon Tartar)

Soups

Bisque (Cream Soup)
Vichyssoise (Potato Leek Soup)

Salads

Artichauts à la Vinaigrette (Artichoke Salad)
Asperge à la Vinaigrette (Asparagus Salad)
Mesclun de Salade (Mixed Green Salad)
Salade Niçoise (Nice Style Salad)

Egg Entrees

Les Oeufs (Fried Eggs)
Les Omelettes (Omelets)

Sample French Menu

Beef Entrees

Filet de Boeuf (Beef Filet)
Fondue Bourguignon (Beef Fondue)
Steak au Poivre (Peppered Steak)
Steak Frites (Steak and French Fried Potatoes)

Chicken Entrees

Poulet Provençal (Roasted Chicken with Herbs)

Seafood Entrees

Bouillabaise (Seafood Stew)
Moules Frites (Mussels and French Fried Potatoes)
Saumon en Papillote (Baked Salmon)

Side Dishes

Gratin Dauphinois (Creamed Potatoes)
Haricots Verts (French Green Beans)
Pommes Frites (French Fried Potatoes)
Ratatouille (Vegetable Stew)

Sample French Menu

Desserts

Assiette de Fromage (Cheese Plate)
Crème Brulée (Baked Custard)
Fruits à la Crème (Fresh Fruit with Cream)
Mousse au Chocolat (Chocolate Mousse)
Les Sorbets (Sorbet)

We would like to thank Nicolas Bergerault, Founder and President of L'atelier des Chefs in Paris, France and Stephane Tremolani, former Executive Chef de Cuisine at the French Embassy in Rome, Italy for their valuable contributions in reviewing the following menu items.

French Menu Item Descriptions

Appetizers
Crevette Cocktail (Shrimp Cocktail)

Shrimp cocktail is a common appetizer across many international cuisines. *Crevette Cocktail* usually refers to medium sized shrimp. *Les Gambas,* large shrimp or prawns, may also be seen on some menus in France. Most restaurants prepare and serve this appetizer in a similar fashion. The shrimp are boiled in water or fish stock, shelled and chilled. They are traditionally served with a cocktail sauce (tomato sauce, horseradish and lemon juice), lemon wedges and sometimes an additional mayonnaise-based sauce.

Gluten-Free Decision Factors:
- Ensure stocks and broths are made fresh and not from bouillon which may contain gluten

- Ensure no wheat flour in sauce

Food Allergen Preparation Considerations:
- Contains shellfish from shrimp

- May contain corn from bouillon and corn syrup in cocktail sauce

- May contain eggs from mayonnaise-based sauce

- May contain fish from fish stock

- May contain soy from bouillon and mayonnaise-based sauce

Escargot (Snails)

Escargot is a delicacy that has been enjoyed in Europe since the time of the ancient Romans. The French have carried on this tradition for hundreds of years and have developed many different recipes for the common garden snail. The texture of prepared escargot is very similar to that of a portabella mushroom and the traditional French preparation is very simple. The snails are removed from the shell and salted for a period of usually three days. Next, a purée of butter, garlic, parsley and shallots is placed in the shell. The snails are returned to the shell and topped with the remainder of the purée. They are then baked and garnished with chopped parsley, pepper and salt before serving. Rather than using shells, some recipes call for mushroom caps or a special ceramic dish to hold the ingredients.

Gluten-Free Decision Factors:
- Ensure no bread crumbs

Food Allergen Preparation Considerations:
- Contains dairy from butter and possibly from bread crumbs
- Contains shellfish from escargot (snails)
- May contain corn from bread crumbs
- May contain eggs from bread crumbs
- May contain peanuts from bread crumbs
- May contain soy from bread crumbs
- May contain tree nuts from bread crumbs

Foies Gras (Fat Liver)
Directly translated *foies gras* or *foie gras* means fat liver. Duck (*le canard*) or goose (*l'oie*) liver is

predominantly used in French cuisine and is served three different ways: whole, in a pâté or in a mousse. French law requires that any product labeled foies gras must be 80% liver, the other 20% can be other meat from chicken, duck, goose or pork. For whole foies gras, the liver is usually marinated overnight in milk or salt water. After being marinated, the liver is thinly sliced, so that all the nerves can be removed. It is then cooked in a terrine with salt, pepper and cognac. Finally, it is set aside for three to four days before being served. Outside of France, you may encounter foies gras that is roasted or pan seared and then served plain or with various vegetables. Pâté de foies gras differs from mousse de foies gras in the consistency of its texture. Both pâté and mousse may contain dairy, eggs and truffles.

Gluten-Free Decision Factors:
- Request no bread

Food Allergen Preparation Considerations:
- May contain corn from bread

- May contain dairy from bread and milk

- May contain eggs as an ingredient and from bread

- May contain peanuts from bread

- May contain soy from bread

- May contain tree nuts from bread

Les Huîtres (Oysters on the Half Shell)

Oysters on the half shell can be served raw with lemon and cocktail sauce. They may also be baked or poached in fresh fish stock and topped with béarnaise or hollandaise sauce.

Gluten-Free Decision Factors:
- Ensure stocks and broths are made fresh and not from bouillon which may contain gluten

- Ensure no wheat flour in sauces

Food Allergen Preparation Considerations:
- Contains shellfish from oysters

- May contain corn from bouillon and corn syrup in cocktail sauce

- May contain dairy from béarnaise and hollandaise sauce

- May contain eggs from béarnaise and hollandaise sauce

- May contain fish from fish stock

- May contain soy from bouillon

Steak Tartare (Beef Tartar)

Steak tartare is a traditional appetizer prepared in French restaurants with many variations. In France, raw ground filet mignon, ground round or ground top sirloin are the common cuts of choice used in this dish. Chopped shallots and capers are served on the side along with lemon, olive oil and white wine vinegar. This allows the guest to pick and choose what ingredients to mix. Outside of France, the dish is usually pre-mixed with the above ingredients and may also include anchovies, garlic and mayonnaise; however, this in uncommon in France. Many recipes also call for a raw egg and white wine. There are a variety of seasonings used including *Herbs de Provence* (marjoram, thyme, summer savory, basil, rosemary, fennel seeds and lavender), mustard powder, pepper and salt. In France, some restaurants may serve Dijon mustard, ketchup (yes, ketchup) and hot pepper sauce on the side.

Gluten-Free Decision Factors:
- None

Food Allergen Preparation Considerations:
- May contain corn from corn syrup in ketchup and vegetable oil
- May contain eggs from mayonnaise and raw egg
- May contain fish from anchovies
- May contain peanuts from vegetable oil
- May contain soy from mayonnaise and vegetable oil

Tartare de Saumon (Salmon Tartar)
There are hundreds of recipes for Salmon Tartar and most are very similar. Raw salmon is either minced or finely cubed. Capers, lemon juice, olive oil, diced scallions and diced shallots are mixed with the salmon and the dish is usually garnished

with fresh dill or parsley. In some regions of France, Dijon mustard or mayonnaise may be included.

Gluten-Free Decision Factors:
- None

Food Allergen Preparation Considerations:
- Contains fish from salmon

- May contain corn from vegetable oil

- May contain eggs from mayonnaise

- May contain peanuts from vegetable oil

- May contain soy from mayonnaise and vegetable oil

Soups
Bisque (Cream Soup)
Bisque is a cream soup that usually features seafood, although vegetable bisques are also common. There are hundreds of recipes for this soup, but most call for standard ingredients. The base of the soup is butter, cream, some type of fresh stock or broth and wine. Onions, puréed tomatoes and potatoes are common vegetables

and the soup can be seasoned with anything from sea salt to saffron. Vegetarian bisques may also include any type of ground nut. Bisques are usually garnished with parsley and sometimes may contain croutons.

Gluten-Free Decision Factors:

- Ensure no croutons

- Ensure no wheat flour as thickening agent

- Ensure stocks and broths are made fresh and not from bouillon which may contain gluten

- Ensure no imitation crabmeat or seafood which may contain gluten

Food Allergen Preparation Considerations:

- Contains dairy from butter and cream

- May contain corn from bouillon and imitation crabmeat

- May contain eggs from croutons and imitation crabmeat

- May contain fish as ingredient and from seafood stock and imitation crabmeat if ordered

- May contain peanuts in vegetable bisque

- May contain shellfish as ingredient and from seafood stock if ordered

- May contain soy from bouillon and imitation crabmeat

- May contain tree nuts in vegetable bisque

Vichyssoise (Potato Leek Soup)

Vichyssoise is a chilled vegetable soup. It was created by Chef Louis Diat at New York's Ritz-Carlton Hotel in 1917, but it is a very common menu item in French restaurants. The base of the soup is butter, fresh chicken broth, cream and white wine. Chives, leeks, onions and potatoes are typically included and the soup is seasoned with basil, bay leaf, chervil, pepper, salt and thyme. The soup is usually garnished with chopped chives or parsley.

Gluten-Free Decision Factors:

- Ensure stocks and broths are made fresh and not from bouillon which may contain gluten

- Ensure no wheat flour as thickening agent

Food Allergen Preparation Considerations:
- Contains dairy from butter and cream
- May contain corn from bouillon
- May contain soy from bouillon

Salads
Artichauts à la Vinaigrette (Artichoke Salad)

Artichokes with vinaigrette are a popular French salad. There are a number of different recipes that either call for whole artichokes or artichoke hearts, which are steamed first to make the meat of the vegetable tender. Of all the different types of vinaigrettes used to dress the artichokes, most usually contain chives, garlic, olive oil, shallots, wine or sherry vinegar and wine. From time to time, you may encounter vinaigrette made with Dijon mustard.

Gluten-Free Decision Factors:
- None

Food Allergen Preparation Considerations:
- May contain corn from vegetable oil

- May contain peanuts from vegetable oil
- May contain soy from vegetable oil

Asperge à la Vinaigrette (Asparagus Salad)

Asparagus with vinaigrette can be prepared many different ways. After the asparagus has been steamed and chilled, chopped onions, tomatoes, shallots and chives can be added. The vinaigrette will usually contain garlic, olive oil, shallots, tarragon, wine or sherry vinegar and wine. From time to time, you may encounter vinaigrette made with Dijon mustard or a vinaigrette that contains hard-boiled eggs.

Gluten-Free Decision Factors:
- None

Food Allergen Preparation Considerations:
- May contain corn from vegetable oil
- May contain eggs from hard-boiled eggs in vinaigrette
- May contain peanuts from vegetable oil
- May contain soy from vegetable oil

Mesclun de Salade (Mixed Green Salad)

Mesclun is a green salad made from several types of young leaves, typically including arugula, dandelion, radicchio, and endive. Some recipes call for fresh berries, carrots, cucumbers, onions, tomatoes, and walnuts. When presented as *Mesclun de Salade*, the dish is usually just the greens tossed in varying types of vinaigrette. From time to time, you may encounter vinaigrette made with Dijon mustard.

Gluten-Free Decision Factors:
- None

Food Allergen Preparation Considerations:
- May contain corn from vegetable oil

- May contain peanuts from vegetable oil

- May contain soy from vegetable oil

- May contain tree nuts from walnuts

Salade Niçoise (Nice Style Salad)

Salade Niçoise comes from the south of France and is a favorite at French restaurants. There are many different recipes, but most usually contain anchovies, hard boiled eggs, green beans, mixed greens, potatoes, olives, onions and tomatoes. Seared tuna is a popular ingredient and you may also encounter salmon. The salad is always accompanied by some type of vinaigrette and may contain Dijon mustard.

Gluten-Free Decision Factors
- None

Food Allergen Preparation Considerations:
- Contains eggs from hard-boiled eggs
- Contains fish from anchovies, salmon or tuna
- May contain corn from vegetable oil
- May contain peanuts from vegetable oil
- May contain soy from vegetable oil

Eggs Entrees
Les Oeufs (Fried Eggs)

Eggs are usually eaten at *le déjeuner* (lunch) and are typically fried in butter in the north of France or olive oil in the south. *Oeuf dur* means "hard boiled eggs," but their consistency in France can sometimes be between soft and hard boiled. Eggs are often accompanied with *jambon* (ham) or *lardon* (fatty bacon).

Gluten-Free Decision Factors:
- Ensure oil used for frying has not been used to fry other items which may be battered or dusted with wheat flour

Food Allergen Preparation Considerations:
- Contains eggs

- May contain corn from vegetable oil

- May contain dairy from butter

- May contain peanuts from peanut oil and vegetable oil

- May contain soy from vegetable oil

Les Omelettes (Omelets)
Omelets are also eaten at *le déjeuner* (lunch) and are usually fried in butter in the north of France or olive oil in the south. Omelets are offered with a variety of ingredients including *nature* (plain),

jambon (ham), *fromage* (cheese), *aux fines herbes* (mixed herbs) and *provençal* (mixed vegetables).

Gluten-Free Decision Factors:
- Ensure oil used for frying has not been used to fry other items which may be battered or dusted with wheat flour

- Ensure no wheat flour as fluffing agent

Food Allergen Preparation Considerations:
- Contains eggs

- May contain corn from vegetable oil

- May contain dairy from butter and cheese

- May contain peanuts from peanut oil and vegetable oil

- May contain soy from vegetable oil

Beef Entrees
Filet de Boeuf (Beef Filet)
Filet de Boeuf is known to most as filet mignon. It is usually seasoned with salt and pepper and may sometimes be seasoned with other herbs. The beef

may be pan seared in butter or olive oil or grilled over an open flame. It is often accompanied with béarnaise or hollandaise sauce. It should be noted that *Filet de Boeuf en Croute,* also known as *Filet de Boeuf Wellington*, is wrapped in puff pastry which contains wheat flour.

Gluten-Free Decision Factors:
- Ensure no wheat flour in sauce

- Ensure beef is not dusted with wheat flour

- Ensure beef is not breaded

Food Allergen Preparation Considerations:
- May contain corn from breading and vegetable oil

- May contain dairy from breading, butter, béarnaise and hollandaise sauce

- May contain eggs from breading, béarnaise and hollandaise sauce

- May contain peanuts from vegetable oil

- May contain soy from breading and vegetable oil

Fondue Bourguignon (Beef Fondue)

Fondue Bourguignon is classic beef fondue. Raw cubes of beef, usually filet mignon or rump steak, are served with a pot of hot vegetable oil. With fondue forks, a diner simply dips the beef into the hot oil until the desired temperature is reached. The dish is accompanied with a variety of dipping sauces and may include béarnaise, hollandaise, mayonnaise and ketchup.

Gluten-Free Decision Factors:

- Ensure no wheat flour in sauce

- Ensure beef is not dusted with wheat flour

Food Allergen Preparation Considerations:

- May contain corn from corn syrup in ketchup and vegetable oil

- May contain dairy from butter, béarnaise and hollandaise sauce

- May contain eggs from mayonnaise, béarnaise and hollandaise sauce

- May contain peanuts from peanut oil and vegetable oil

- May contain soy from mayonnaise and vegetable oil

Steak au Poivre (Peppered Steak)

Steak au Poivre is a standard French beef dish. Strip or sirloin steak is salted and pan fried with a little olive oil or butter. The French prefer the cooking temperature to be rare (bleu) or medium rare (à point). The steak is removed and a reduction of butter, red wine and cracked peppercorn is made in the pan using the fat or jus that remains. Garlic and shallots are sometimes used in the sauce. The dish is usually served with a side of *haricots verts* (French green beans) and carrots.

Gluten-Free Decision Factors:
- Ensure no wheat flour in sauce
- Ensure beef is not dusted with wheat flour

Food Allergen Preparation Considerations:
- Contains dairy from butter
- May contain corn from vegetable oil
- May contain peanuts from vegetable oil
- May contain soy from vegetable oil

Steak Frites (Steak and French Fried Potatoes)

Steak Frites can be many cuts of meat including porterhouse, sirloin, rib eye, shell steak or filet mignon. The steak is usually pan fried in butter or oil and seasoned with salt and pepper. Once the steak is done, a reduction can be made with butter, shallots and red wine. The steak is always accompanied by *pommes frites* (French fried potatoes) and may come with herb butter, ketchup, mayonnaise, béarnaise or hollandaise sauce. Malt vinegar is a common table condiment used for *pommes frites* in French restaurants and contains gluten.

Gluten-Free Decision Factors:

- Ensure no wheat flour in sauce

- Ensure beef is not dusted with wheat flour

- Ensure potatoes are not dusted with wheat flour

- Ensure oil used for frying is designated for potatoes only and is not used to fry other items that may be battered or dusted with wheat flour

- Request no malt vinegar

Food Allergen Preparation Considerations:

- May contain corn from corn syrup in ketchup and vegetable oil

- May contain dairy from butter, béarnaise and hollandaise sauce

- May contain eggs from mayonnaise, béarnaise and hollandaise sauce

- May contain peanuts from peanut oil and vegetable oil

- May contain soy from mayonnaise and vegetable oil

Chicken Entrees
Poulet Provençal (Roasted Chicken with Herbs)

Poulet Provençal is a marinated chicken dish that is either roasted in a special rotisserie oven or baked. This dish is a variation of the ubiquitous *Poulet Roti* (roasted chicken) found all over France. The whole chicken is marinated with garlic, *Herbs de Provence* (marjoram, thyme, summer savory, basil, rosemary, fennel seeds and lavender), lemon juice, olive oil, pepper and salt. After it is roasted, the chicken is served with vegetables which may include roasted potatoes with rosemary and salt or *haricots verts* (French green beans).

Gluten-Free Decision Factors:
- Ensure no soy sauce or wheat flour in marinade

Food Allergen Preparation Considerations:
- May contain dairy from butter in side vegetables

- May contain soy from soy sauce in marinade

- May contain tree nuts in side vegetables

Seafood Entrees
Bouillabaise (Seafood Stew)
More than just a soup or stew, *Bouillabaise* is a French gastronomic tradition. In a clear fresh fish stock or broth, many types of seafood are combined including clams, crab, any fish, lobster, mussels, oysters, scallops and shrimp. The vegetables usually included are carrots, celery, leeks, onions and potatoes. *Bouillabaise* is typically seasoned with garlic, pepper, salt and saffron, but may also be sea-

soned with a *bouquet garni* (cheese cloth bag full of herbs) containing *Herbes de Provence*. Some recipes call for croutons or toasted bread on the side.

Gluten-Free Decision Factors:
- Ensure no croutons or bread
- Ensure no wheat flour as thickening agent
- Ensure stocks or broths are made fresh and not from bouillon which may contain gluten

Food Allergen Preparation Considerations:
- Contains fish as an ingredient
- Contains shellfish as an ingredient
- May contain corn from bouillon and bread
- May contain dairy from bread
- May contain eggs from bread and croutons
- May contain peanuts from bread
- May contain soy from bouillon and bread
- May contain tree nuts from bread

Moules Frites (Mussels and French Fried Potatoes)

Steamed mussels are very popular in Belgium and France. They are served both as an appetizer and as an entrée and are typically accompanied with *pommes frites*. The mussels are steamed or boiled in fresh fish stock, then topped with a sauce that contains butter, onions or shallots, white wine and sometimes garlic. Occasionally, the mussels may be topped with bread crumbs. *Pommes frites* may come with herb butter, ketchup, mayonnaise, béarnaise or hollandaise sauce. Malt vinegar is a common table condiment used for *pommes frites* in French restaurants and contains gluten.

Gluten-Free Decision Factors:

- Ensure no wheat flour in sauce

- Ensure no bread crumbs

- Ensure stocks and broths are made fresh and not from bouillon which may contain gluten

- Ensure potatoes are not dusted with wheat flour

- Ensure oil used for frying is designated for potatoes only and is not used to fry other items that may be battered or dusted with wheat flour

- Request no malt vinegar

Food Allergen Preparation Considerations:
- Contains dairy from butter and possibly from bread crumbs, béarnaise and hollandaise sauce

- Contains shellfish from mussels

- May contain corn from bouillon, bread crumbs, corn syrup in ketchup and vegetable oil

- May contain eggs from bread crumbs, mayonnaise, béarnaise and hollandaise sauce

- May contain peanuts from bread crumbs, peanut oil and vegetable oil

- May contain soy from bouillon, bread crumbs and vegetable oil

- May contain tree nuts from bread crumbs

Saumon en Papillote (Baked Salmon)

The term *"en Papillote"* refers to the French style of cooking in a parchment paper bag. This is an excellent way to cook, as it allows all the flavors inside to permeate the fish. You may find any fish made *"en Papillote."* A filet of salmon is placed in the center of a large piece of parchment paper that has been brushed with butter or olive oil. Blanched vegetables including julienned carrots, leeks and green beans are added to garlic, onions and shallots that are sautéed in butter or olive oil. The dish can be seasoned with various herbs including coriander, fennel, pepper and salt. The parchment paper is then folded in the shape of a bag and baked until brown. Egg whites are sometimes used to seal the parchment paper bag.

Gluten-Free Decision Factors:
• Ensure fish is not dusted with wheat flour

Food Allergen Preparation Considerations:
• Contains fish from salmon

• May contain corn from vegetable oil

• May contain dairy from butter

- May contain eggs from the sealing of parchment paper bag

- May contain peanuts from peanut oil and vegetable oil

- May contain soy from vegetable oil

Side Dishes
Gratin Dauphinois (Creamed Potatoes)

A creamed potato casserole, *Gratin Dauphinois* is a common French side dish. Thinly sliced potatoes are baked in a cream sauce with butter, crème fraîche and milk. It is seasoned with garlic, salt, pepper and may also contain nutmeg. Some recipes call for grated gruyère cheese and bread crumbs; however the traditional style omits these ingredients.

Gluten-Free Decision Factors:
- Ensure no wheat flour as ingredient

- Ensure no bread crumbs

Food Allergen Preparation Considerations:
- Contains dairy from butter, crème fraîche, milk and possibly from bread crumbs and cheese

- May contain corn from bread crumbs

- May contain eggs from bread crumbs

- May contain peanuts from bread crumbs

- May contain soy from bread crumbs

- May contain tree nuts from bread crumbs

Haricots Verts (French Green Beans)

The French prepare green beans by steaming them until they are cooked, yet still crisp. *Haricots verts* can be served plain, in butter or olive oil and may contain almonds, garlic and onions. They may also be topped with béarnaise or hollandaise sauce.

Gluten-Free Decision Factors:

- Ensure no wheat flour in sauce

Food Allergen Preparation Considerations:

- May contain corn from vegetable oil

- May contain dairy from butter, béarnaise or hollandaise sauce

- May contain eggs from béarnaise or hollandaise sauce

- May contain peanuts from peanut oil and vegetable oil

- May contain soy from vegetable oil

- May contain tree nuts from almonds

Pommes Frites (French Fried Potatoes)

Pommes Frites are classic French fried potatoes, although many give credit to the Belgians for creating this dish. The potatoes are typically sliced very thin and fried in peanut or vegetable oil. They are seasoned with salt, but some recipes call for a butter, garlic and parsley sauce on the side for dipping. The French also like to dip them in herb butter, ketchup, mayonnaise, béarnaise or hollandaise sauce. Malt vinegar is a common table condiment used for *pommes frites* in French restaurants and contains gluten.

Gluten-Free Decision Factors:

- Ensure potatoes are not dusted with wheat flour prior to frying

- Ensure oil used for frying is designated for potatoes only and is not used to fry other items that may be battered or dusted with wheat flour

- Request no malt vinegar

Food Allergen Preparation Considerations:
- May contain corn from corn syrup in ketchup and vegetable oil

- May contain dairy from butter, béarnaise and hollandaise sauce

- May contain eggs from mayonnaise, béarnaise and hollandaise sauce

- May contain peanuts from peanut oil and vegetable oil

- May contain soy from mayonnaise and vegetable oil

Ratatouille (Vegetable Stew)

Ratatouille is a traditional vegetable dish from the south of France that can be served as a side dish as well as an entrée. It resembles a vegetable stew and includes bell peppers, eggplant, onions, tomatoes and zucchini. The vegetables are cooked in olive oil and white wine, then seasoned with garlic, *Herbs de Provence*, pepper and salt. Although uncommon, some recipes call for grated cheese. *Ratatouille* can be served hot or chilled.

Gluten-Free Decision Factors:
- Ensure no wheat flour as ingredient
- Ensure stocks and broths are made fresh and not from bouillon which may contain gluten

Food Allergen Preparation Considerations:
- May contain corn from bouillon and vegetable oil
- May contain dairy from cheese
- May contain peanuts from vegetable oil
- May contain soy from bouillon and vegetable oil

Desserts
Assiette de Fromage (Cheese Plate)
Generally speaking, cheese is eaten with salad prior to the dessert course in France and is typically listed in the dessert section of the menu. In most cases, you

are offered a variety of different cheeses including brie, camembert and chèvre; however, the types may vary based upon location and availability. Cheese is usually served with bread or crackers and sometimes sliced fruit.

Gluten-Free Decision Factors:
- Request no bread or crackers
- Request no blue or veined cheese which may contain gluten

Food Allergen Preparation Considerations:
- Contains dairy from cheese and possibly from bread
- May contain corn from bread
- May contain eggs as ingredient and from bread
- May contain peanuts from bread
- May contain soy from bread
- May contain tree nuts from bread

Crème Brulée (Baked Custard)

Crème Brulée is one of the most popular French desserts. The custard is made with heavy cream, egg yolks, sugar and vanilla. The whisked ingredients are then baked. After it has cooled, it is topped with brown sugar that is caramelized by placing the custard in a broiler or torching it by hand. There are many different types of crème brulée, some of which may contain different flavors such as almond, chocolate and fresh berries.

Gluten-Free Decision Factors:

- Ensure no wheat flour as ingredient

Food Allergen Preparation Considerations:

- Contains dairy from cream

- Contains eggs from egg yolks

- May contain corn from almond and vanilla extract

- May contain soy from chocolate

- May contain tree nuts from almond extract

Fruits à la Crème (Fresh Fruit with Cream)

Crème fraîche is a slightly tangy and nutty thick cream that is naturally fermented. The French adore this cream as a dessert with fresh fruit. Mixed berries are usually the fruit of choice, but you can find it with other fruits such as apples and melons.

Gluten-Free Decision Factors:
- None

Food Allergen Preparation Considerations:
- Contains dairy from cream

Mousse au Chocolat (Chocolate Mousse)

Chocolate mousse has become a popular dessert and can be found on the menus of many international cuisines. There are a number of variations, but the preparation is typically consistent with the following recipe. Chocolate is melted in a double-boiler with milk and sugar. Whipped eggs are then carefully folded into the chocolate sauce after it has cooled. Next, whipped heavy cream is added to the mixture, which is allowed to sit for a few minutes before the mousse is poured into a container and chilled. Some styles incorporate liqueurs such as coffee, orange and peppermint for a distinctive flavor. Chocolate mousse may be served with whipped cream and a cookie.

Gluten-Free Decision Factors:
- Ensure no wheat flour as ingredient
- Request no cookie

Food Allergen Preparation Considerations:
- Contains dairy from cream, milk and possibly from chocolate and cookie
- Contains eggs as an ingredient and possibly from cookie
- May contain peanuts from cookie and various flavors
- May contain tree nuts from cookie and various flavors

Les Sorbets (Sorbet)
Sorbet is puréed fruit and sugar that is frozen and served like ice cream. If the restaurant uses *service à la russe*, sorbet may be offered in between courses

to cleanse your palate. Raspberry, lemon and lime sorbets are the most common. You may also encounter many other fruit flavors or chocolate. Occasionally, sorbet is served with some kind of cookie or pirouline.

Gluten-Free Decision Factors:
- Ensure no wheat flour as ingredient
- Ensure no stabilizers which may contain gluten
- Request no cookie

Food Allergen Preparation Considerations:
- May contain corn from colors or flavors
- May contain dairy from cookie
- May contain eggs from cookie
- May contain peanuts from cookie and various flavors
- May contain soy from chocolate, colors or flavors and cookie
- May contain tree nuts from cookie and various flavors

French Cuisine:
Quick Reference Guide
(Appetizers – Soups)

	Corn	Dairy	Eggs	Fish	Gluten/Wheat	Peanuts	Shellfish	Soy	Tree Nuts
Appetizers									
Crevette Cocktail (Shrimp Cocktail)	O		O	O	O		●	O	
Escargot (Snails)	O	●	O		O	O	●	O	O
Foies Gras (Fat Liver)	O	O	O		O	O		O	O
Les Huîtres (Oysters on the Half Shell)	O	O	O	O	O		●	O	
Steak Tartare (Beef Tartar)	O		O	O		O		O	
Tartare de Saumon (Salmon Tartar)	O		O	●		O		O	
Soups									
Bisque (Cream Soup)	O	●	O	O	O	O	O	O	O
Vichyssoise (Potato Leek Soup)	O	●			O			O	

Always ensure no cross-contamination in food preparation

● Typically contains allergen   O May contain allergen

French Cuisine:
Quick Reference Guide
(Salads – Egg Entrees)

	Corn	Dairy	Eggs	Fish	Gluten/Wheat	Peanuts	Shellfish	Soy	Tree Nuts
Salads									
Artichauts à la Vinaigrette (Artichoke Salad)	O					O		O	
Asperge à la Vinaigrette (Asparagus Salad)	O		O			O		O	
Mesclun de Salade (Mixed Green Salad)	O					O		O	O
Salade Niçoise (Nice Style Salad)	O		●	●		O		O	
Egg Entrees									
Les Oeufs (Fried Eggs)	O	O	●		O	O		O	
Les Omelettes (Omelets)	O	O	●		O	O		O	

Always ensure no cross-contamination in food preparation

● Typically contains allergen   O May contain allergen

French Cuisine:
Quick Reference Guide
(Beef Entrees – Chicken Entrees)

	Corn	Dairy	Eggs	Fish	Gluten/Wheat	Peanuts	Shellfish	Soy	Tree Nuts
Beef Entrees									
Filet de Boeuf (Beef Filet)	O	O	O		O	O		O	
Fondue Bourguignon (Beef Fondue)	O	O	O		O	O		O	
Steak au Poivre (Peppered Steak)	O	●			O	O		O	
Steak Frites (Steak and French Fried Potatoes)	O	O	O		O	O		O	
Chicken Entrees									
Poulet Provençal (Roasted Chicken with Herbs)		O			O			O	O

Always ensure no cross-contamination in food preparation

● Typically contains allergen   O May contain allergen

French Cuisine: Quick Reference Guide

(Seafood Entrees – Side Dishes)

	Corn	Dairy	Eggs	Fish	Gluten/Wheat	Peanuts	Shellfish	Soy	Tree Nuts
Seafood Entrees									
Bouillabaise (Seafood Stew)	O	O	O	●	O		●	O	O
Moules Frites (Mussels and French Fried Potatoes)	O	●	O	O	O	O	●	O	O
Saumon en Papillote (Baked Salmon)	O	O	O	●	O	O		O	
Side Dishes									
Gratin Dauphinois (Creamed Potatoes)	O	●	O		O	O		O	O
Haricots Verts (French Green Beans)	O	O	O		O	O		O	O
Pommes Frites (French Fried Potatoes)	O	O	O		O	O		O	
Ratatouille (Vegetable Stew)	O	O			O	O		O	

Always ensure no cross-contamination in food preparation

● Typically contains allergen   O May contain allergen

French Cuisine:
Quick Reference Guide
(Desserts)

Desserts	Corn	Dairy	Eggs	Fish	Gluten/Wheat	Peanuts	Shellfish	Soy	Tree Nuts
Assiette de Fromage (Cheese Plate)	O	●	O		O	O		O	O
Crème Brulée (Baked Custard)	O	●	●		O			O	O
Fruits à la Crème (Fresh Fruit with Cream)		●							
Mousse au Chocolat (Chocolate Mousse)	O	●	●		O	O		O	O
Les Sorbets (Sorbet)	O	O	O		O	O		O	O

Always ensure no cross-contamination in food preparation

● Typically contains allergen   O May contain allergen

58

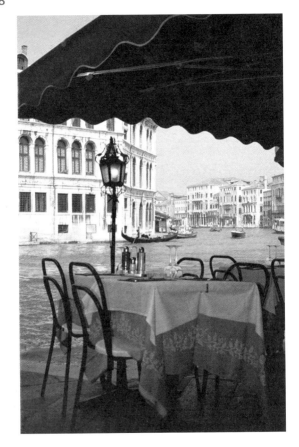

One of the very nicest things about life
is the way we must regularly stop whatever it is
we are doing and devote our attention to eating.
—Luciano Pavarotti

Let's Eat Italian Cuisine

Cuisine Overview

The following materials outline:

- Dining considerations
- Sample Italian menu
- Italian cuisine menu items and descriptions
- Quick reference guide

Dining Considerations

Italian menu items are usually presented in the Italian language. You may often find menu descriptions in the language of the country you are in following the name of the Italian menu item. While traveling, be sure to familiarize yourself with the common Italian culinary terms included in this chapter to assist you in your dining experience.

Italians generally eat two meals a day. In the morning, they usually drink coffee with warm milk and may have a *biscotti* or sweet biscuit. The first big meal of the day happens between 1 p.m. and 3 p.m. and is called *pranzo*. This is usually the largest meal of the day and consists of four to five courses. The evening meal or *cena* is usually a quick affair when eaten at home with the family, beginning at 8 p.m. and ending before nine. As a special meal, *cena* can be enjoyed later than many people are used to, sometimes beginning at 9 or 10 p.m. It is a lighter meal than the afternoon *pranzo*. When dining out or entertaining guests in the home, Italians like to eat slowly and savor their food. Most meals typically last between two to three hours. Wine and conversation are a must at an Italian table, so it is best to relax and enjoy the experience.

There are generally four courses to a meal: *antipasto* (soups, salads or appetizers), *primo* (pasta), *secondo* (entrées) and *dolce* (desserts). Occasionally, an additional vegetable course may be added after the *secondo* and is called the *contorno*. Wine is served continually throughout the meal, with sweet dessert wines enjoyed at the end of the meal.

Buon Appetito!

Sample Italian Menu

Appetizers

Calamari alla Griglia (Grilled Calamari)
Carpaccio di Manzo (Beef Carpaccio)
Carpaccio di Salmone (Salmon Carpaccio)
Cocktail di Gamberi (Shrimp Cocktail)
Cozze al Vapore (Steamed Mussels)
Prosciutto e Melone (Cured Ham and Melon)

Soups

Gazpaccio

Salads

Insalata Caprese (Mozzarella Tomato Salad)
Insalata Mista (Mixed Green Salad)

Italian Specialties

Risotto ai Frutti di Mare (Arborio Rice & Seafood Dish)
Risotto ai Funghi (Arborio Rice & Mushroom Dish)
Risotto ai Quattro Formaggi (Arborio Rice & Cheese Dish)
Risotto al Pollo (Arborio Rice & Chicken Dish)

Sample Italian Menu

Meat Entrees

Costatella D'Agnello (Rack of Lamb)
Fileto di Manzo (Filet Mignon)
Medalione di Manzo (Beef Tenderloin Medallions)
Vitello (Veal)

Chicken Entrees

Petti di Pollo (Chicken Breast)
Pollo Arrosto Rosmarino (Rosemary Roasted Chicken)

Seafood Entrees

Salmone alla Griglia (Grilled Salmon)
Scampi (Prawns)

Side Dishes

Broccoli Rabe (Broccoli Florets)
Funghi all' Aglio e Olio (Mushrooms in Garlic & Olive Oil)
Melanzane alla Griglia (Grilled Eggplant)
Polenta (Boiled Corn Meal)

Desserts

Frutti di Stagione (Fresh Fruit in Season)
Gelato (Italian Ice Cream or Sherbet)
Granita (Italian Ice)
Zabaglione (Italian Custard)

We would like to thank Arber Murici of Lumi in New York, New York and Stephane Tremolani, former Executive Chef de Cuisine of the French Embassy in Rome, Italy for their valuable contributions in reviewing the following menu items.

Italian Menu Item Descriptions

Appetizers
Calamari alla Griglia (Grilled Calamari)

Many Italian restaurants offer grilled calamari; however, it is more commonly fried. Slices of calamari are marinated in lemon juice or olive oil then cooked on a grill over an open flame. Lemon wedges and marinara sauce for dipping are usually served on the side.

Gluten-Free Decision Factors:

- Ensure no wheat flour in sauce

- Ensure calamari is not battered

- Ensure calamari is not dusted with wheat flour

- Ensure no bread crumbs

Food Allergen Preparation Considerations:

- Contains shellfish from calamari

- May contain corn from batter, bread crumbs, dipping sauce and vegetable oil

- May contain dairy from bread crumbs and dipping sauce

- May contain eggs from batter, bread crumbs and dipping sauce

- May contain peanuts from bread crumbs, dipping sauce and vegetable oil

- May contain soy from bread crumbs and vegetable oil

- May contain tree nuts from bread crumbs and dipping sauce

Carpaccio di Manzo (Beef Carpaccio)

Beef Carpaccio is thinly sliced rare beef lightly dressed with olive oil and sometimes balsamic vinegar. Shaved *parmigiano reggiano,* capers and dried herbs top the beef. This dish is generally garnished with fresh basil.

Gluten-Free Decision Factors:
- None

Food Allergen Preparation Considerations:
- Contains dairy from cheese

- May contain corn from vegetable oil

- May contain peanuts from vegetable oil

- May contain soy from vegetable oil

Carpaccio di Salmone (Salmon Carpaccio)

Like Beef Carpaccio, Salmon Carpaccio is thinly sliced raw salmon marinated in olive oil and lemon. There are many different recipes for this dish, however they are all similar. In some variations, balsamic vinegar, shallots, fresh dill and capers can be present. You may encounter a version of *Carpaccio di Salmone* at a restaurant that includes fava beans. The preparation of the fava beans most likely contains wheat flour.

Gluten-Free Decision Factors:
- Ensure no wheat flour in fava beans

Food Allergen Preparation Considerations:
- Contains fish from salmon
- May contain corn from vegetable oil
- May contain corn from vegetable oil
- May contain soy from vegetable oil

Cocktail di Gamberi (Shrimp Cocktail)

Shrimp cocktail is a common appetizer in many international cuisines. Most restaurants prepare and serve this appetizer in a similar fashion. Large shrimp are boiled in water or fish stock, shelled and chilled. The shrimp are served with a cocktail sauce (tomato sauce, horseradish and lemon juice) and lemon wedges. Italians prefer a mayonnaise-based cocktail sauce made with ketchup, a dash of pepper sauce and a touch of liquor such as whiskey or cognac.

Gluten-Free Decision Factors:
- Ensure stocks and broths are made fresh and not from bouillon which may contain gluten

Food Allergen Preparation Considerations:
- Contains shellfish from shrimp

- May contain corn from bouillon and corn syrup in cocktail sauce

- May contain eggs from mayonnaise-based sauce

- May contain fish from fish stock

- May contain soy from bouillon and mayonnaise-based sauce

Cozze al Vapore (Steamed Mussels)

Steamed mussels are a very popular appetizer in Italian restaurants. They are served both as an appetizer or as an entrée, which is usually accompanied with pasta. The mussels are steamed or boiled in fish stock, then topped with a sauce that contains butter, onions or shallots, white wine and sometimes garlic. Occasionally, the mussels may be topped with bread crumbs.

Gluten-Free Decision Factors:

- Ensure no bread crumbs

- Ensure no wheat flour pasta—order gluten-free pasta or polenta if available

- Ensure stocks and broths are made fresh and not from bouillon which may contain gluten

Food Allergen Preparation Considerations:

- Contains dairy from butter and possibly from bread crumbs

- Contains shellfish from mussels

- May contain corn from bouillon and bread crumbs

- May contain eggs from bread crumbs and pasta

- May contain peanuts from bread crumbs

- May contain soy from bread crumbs and bouillon

- May contain tree nuts from bread crumbs

Prosciutto e Melone (Cured Ham and Melon)

Prosciutto e Melone is a common dish found in many Italian restaurants. It is fresh cantaloupe or honey dew wrapped with *prosciutto di parma*, an Italian cured ham. Sometimes the dish contains aged hard cheese such as *parmigiano reggiano*.

Gluten-Free Decision Factors:
- None

Food Allergen Preparation Considerations:
- May contain dairy from cheese

Soups
Gazpaccio

This chilled soup usually consists of puréed tomatoes, onions, peppers and garlic, but may contain any fresh vegetable. It is seasoned with salt and pepper and may also contain other fresh Italian herbs. The popularity of gazpaccio has allowed this soup to be adapted into many regional cuisines in Europe. Although it is uncommon in Italy, restaurants outside the country may add wheat flour and croutons.

Gluten-Free Decision Factors:
- Ensure no croutons

- Ensure no wheat flour as thickening agent

Food Allergen Preparation Considerations:
- May contain corn as ingredient

- May contain eggs from croutons

Salads

Insalata Caprese (Mozzarella Tomato Salad)

Buffalo mozzarella and tomato salad is an Italian classic. Large slices of buffalo mozzarella are stacked with freshly sliced tomatoes. It is usually seasoned with salt and pepper and potentially other dried herbs on occasion. Large leafs of basil garnish this dish, which is lightly dressed in olive oil and sometimes balsamic vinegar.

Gluten-Free Decision Factors:
- None

Food Allergen Preparation Considerations:
- Contains dairy from cheese

- May contain corn from vegetable oil

- May contain peanuts from vegetable oil

- May contain soy from vegetable oil

Insalata Mista (Mixed Green Salad)

A mixed green salad in Italy is usually a combination of mixed greens, cucumbers, onions and tomatoes. Some Italian restaurants may add anchovies or croutons and the type of salad dressings may vary.

Gluten-Free Decision Factors:
- Request no croutons

Food Allergen Preparation Considerations:
- May contain corn from vegetable oil
- May contain eggs from croutons
- May contain fish from anchovies
- May contain peanuts from vegetable oil
- May contain soy from vegetable oil

Italian Specialties
Risotto ai Frutti di Mare (Arborio Rice and Seafood Dish)

Risotto is a Northern Italian dish with seafood being one of the common varieties. The preparation techniques of *risotto* dishes are usually similar, but the ingredients vary depending on the type of *risotto* that you order. In *Risotto ai Frutti di Mare,* arborio rice is boiled in fresh stock, usually chicken, fish or shrimp. In a separate pan, white wine is simmered with garlic, olive oil, onions or shallots, salt and pepper. Mushrooms such as porcini or portabella are often added. Mixed seafood (usually calamari, clams, fish, oysters, mussels, scallops and shrimp) is then cooked in the wine until its temperature is somewhere between rare and medium rare. The seafood is then added to the rice, which has had fresh stock continually added to it as the moisture evaporates. As the moisture continues to evaporate, butter, *parmigiano reggiano* and *romano* cheese are added. The dish is usually garnished with parsley.

Gluten-Free Decision Factors:
- Ensure stocks and broths are made fresh and not from bouillon which may contain gluten

Food Allergen Preparation Considerations:
- Contains dairy from butter and cheese
- Contains fish as ingredient
- Contains shellfish as ingredient
- May contain corn from bouillon and vegetable oil
- May contain peanuts from vegetable oil

- May contain soy from bouillon and vegetable oil

Risotto ai Funghi (Arborio Rice and Mushroom Dish)

In *Risotto ai Funghi,* arborio rice is boiled in fresh stock, usually chicken or mushroom. In a separate pan, white wine is simmered with garlic, olive oil, onions or shallots, salt and pepper. Mushrooms such as cremini, porcini and portabella are added. Some recipes may even call for *tartufi,* which are black or white truffles. The mushrooms are then added to the rice, which has had fresh stock continually added to it as the moisture evaporates. As the moisture continues to evaporate, butter, *parmigiano reggiano* and *romano* cheese are added. The dish is usually garnished with parsley.

Gluten-Free Decision Factors:

- Ensure stocks and broths are made fresh and not from bouillon which may contain gluten

Food Allergen Preparation Considerations:

- Contains dairy from butter and cheese

- May contain corn from bouillon and vegetable oil

- May contain peanuts from vegetable oil
- May contain soy from bouillon and vegetable oil

Risotto ai Quattro Formaggi (Arborio Rice and Cheese Dish)

In *Risotto ai Quattro Formaggi,* arborio rice is boiled in fresh stock, usually chicken or vegetable. In a separate pan, white wine is simmered with garlic, olive oil, onions or shallots, salt and pepper. This is then added to the rice, which has had fresh stock continually added to it as the moisture evaporates. As the moisture continues to evaporate, butter, *fontina, parmigiano reggiano, pecorino* and *romano* cheese are added. The dish is usually garnished with parsley.

Gluten-Free Decision Factors:
- Ensure stocks and broths are made fresh and not from bouillon which may contain gluten

Food Allergen Preparation Considerations:
- Contains dairy from butter and cheese
- May contain corn from bouillon and vegetable oil

- May contain peanuts from vegetable oil

- May contain soy from bouillon and vegetable
  oil

Risotto al Pollo (Arborio Rice and Chicken Dish)

In *Risotto al Pollo,* arborio rice is boiled in fresh
chicken stock. In a separate pan, white wine is
simmered with garlic, olive oil, onions or shallots,
salt and pepper. Slices of chicken are then added,
sometimes with aromatic herbs such as anise, fennel or rosemary. The chicken is then added to the
rice, which had fresh stock continually added
to it as the moisture evaporates. As the moisture
continues to evaporate, butter, *parmigiano reggiano*
and *romano* cheese are added. The dish is usually
garnished with parsley.

Gluten-Free Decision Factors:

- Ensure stocks and broths are made fresh and
  not from bouillon which may contain gluten

Food Allergen Preparation Considerations:

- Contains dairy from butter and cheese

- May contain corn from bouillon and vegetable oil

- May contain peanuts from vegetable oil

- May contain soy from bouillon and vegetable oil

Meat Entrees
Costatella D'Agnello (Rack of Lamb)

Costatella (rack) or *costoletta* (chop) are widely considered the most flavorful cut of lamb. They are taken from the rib and have a good amount of marbling, which provides the rich flavor. Italians traditionally roast lamb with olive oil, rosemary, salt, pepper and plenty of garlic. If the menu description states that the dish is herb encrusted, bread crumbs are usually used. The dish is typically served with a side vegetable or pasta.

Gluten-Free Decision Factors:

- Ensure lamb is not dusted with wheat flour

- Ensure no wheat flour pasta—order gluten-free pasta or polenta if available

- Ensure no bread crumbs

Food Allergen Preparation Considerations:

- Food allergens may vary in side vegetables

- May contain corn from bread crumbs and vegetable oil

- May contain dairy from bread crumbs

- May contain eggs from bread crumbs and pasta

- May contain peanuts from bread crumbs and vegetable oil

- May contain soy from bread crumbs and vegetable oil

- May contain tree nuts from bread crumbs

Fileto di Manzo (Filet Mignon)

Fileto di Manzo is the classic dish known to most as filet mignon. It is usually seasoned with salt and pepper and may sometimes be seasoned with other Italian herbs. The beef may be pan seared in butter or olive oil; it can also be grilled over an open flame. The dish is typically served with a side vegetable or pasta.

Gluten-Free Decision Factors:
- Ensure beef is not dusted with wheat flour
- Ensure no wheat flour pasta—order gluten-free pasta or polenta if available

Food Allergen Preparation Considerations:
- Food allergens may vary in side vegetables
- May contain corn from vegetable oil
- May contain dairy from butter
- May contain eggs from pasta
- May contain peanuts from vegetable oil
- May contain soy from vegetable oil

Medalione di Manzo (Beef Tenderloin Medallions)
Slices of beef tenderloin are pan seared in butter or olive oil, or they can be grilled over an open flame. The medallions are usually seasoned with salt and pepper and may also be seasoned with other Italian herbs. It is common for the medallions to be served in *marinara* or *pomodoro* sauce. The dish is typically served with a side vegetable or pasta.

Gluten-Free Decision Factors:
- Ensure no wheat flour in sauce

- Ensure beef is not dusted with wheat flour

- Ensure no wheat flour pasta—order gluten-free pasta or polenta if available

Other Potential Allergens
- Food allergens may vary in side vegetables

- May contain corn from vegetable oil

- May contain dairy from butter and sauce

- May contain eggs from pasta

- May contain peanuts from vegetable oil

- May contain soy from vegetable oil

- May contain tree nuts from sauce

Vitello (Veal)

Veal is a very popular type of meat served in Italian restaurants. It is meat from a young calf, usually eight months in age, and considered more tender and flavorful than regular beef. The most common cuts of veal you may encounter are *scallopine* (cutlet), *costatella* (rack of rib) and *costoletta* (chop). Veal can be prepared a number of different ways and is usually grilled, pan seared or roasted. When offered as *scallopine,* it is typically served in a sauce like *parmigiana* (a tomato sauce with *parmigiano reggiano* cheese) or *piccata* (a lemon and caper sauce made with white wine and butter). In the case of *parmigiana* or *piccata*, the veal may be breaded or flour dusted. If the menu description states that the veal is herb encrusted, bread crumbs are typically used. Veal is usually served with a side vegetable or pasta in restaurants outside of Italy. However, pasta with veal in Italy is uncommon.

Gluten-Free Decision Factors:

- Ensure no wheat flour in sauce

- Ensure no breading

- Ensure veal is not dusted with wheat flour

- Ensure no bread crumbs

- Ensure no wheat flour pasta—order gluten-free pasta or polenta if available

Food Allergen Preparation Considerations:

- Food allergens may vary in side vegetables

- May contain corn from bread crumbs, breading and vegetable oil

- May contain dairy from bread crumbs, breading, butter, cheese and sauce

- May contain eggs from bread crumbs, breading and pasta

- May contain peanuts from bread crumbs and vegetable oil

- May contain soy from bread crumbs, breading and vegetable oil

- May contain tree nuts from bread crumbs and sauce

Chicken Entrees
Petti di Pollo (Chicken Breast)

Grilled chicken breast is a relatively common menu item in Italian restaurants. Chicken breasts can be prepared many different ways and usually come topped with a sauce. Some chicken breast entrées with sauces include; *all' anice* (a cream sauce with anise and fennel), *al limone* (*piccata* style in a lemon and caper sauce made with white wine and butter) and *parmigiana*. In the case of *al limone* or *parmigiana*, the chicken may be breaded or flour dusted. If the menu description states that the chicken is herb encrusted, bread crumbs are typically used. Chicken breast entrées are usually accompanied by a side vegetable or pasta.

Gluten-Free Decision Factors:
- Ensure no wheat flour in sauce
- Ensure no breading
- Ensure chicken is not dusted with wheat flour
- Ensure no bread crumbs
- Ensure no wheat flour pasta—order gluten-free pasta or polenta if available

Food Allergen Preparation Considerations:
- Food allergens may vary in side vegetables
- May contain corn from bread crumbs, breading and vegetable oil
- May contain dairy from bread crumbs, breading, butter, cheese, cream and sauce
- May contain eggs from bread crumbs, breading and pasta

- May contain peanuts from bread crumbs and vegetable oil

- May contain soy from bread crumbs, breading and vegetable oil

- May contain tree nuts from bread crumbs and sauce

Pollo Arrosto Rosmarino (Rosemary Roasted Chicken)

Italian restaurants serve many different styles of roasted chicken, with rosemary being the most commonly used herb. A whole chicken is rubbed with olive oil, fresh rosemary, salt, pepper and possibly anise, fennel, garlic, oregano and thyme. It is then roasted in an oven or over an open flame. Half a roasted chicken is the common portion. If the menu description states that the chicken is herb encrusted, bread crumbs are typically used. The dish is usually served with a side vegetable or pasta.

Gluten-Free Decision Factors:

- Ensure no bread crumbs

- Ensure no wheat flour pasta—order gluten-free pasta or polenta if available

Food Allergen Preparation Considerations:

- Food allergens may vary in side vegetables

- May contain corn from bread crumbs and vegetable oil

- May contain dairy from bread crumbs

- May contain eggs from bread crumbs and pasta

- May contain peanuts from bread crumbs and vegetable oil

- May contain soy from bread crumbs and vegetable oil

- May contain tree nuts from bread crumbs

Seafood Entrees
Salmone alla Griglia (Grilled Salmon)

Grilled salmon is popular in Italian restaurants in the coastal areas of Italy, as well outside of the country. Salmon filets are grilled and seasoned with fresh lemon juice and herbs, usually dill or rosemary. Once cooked, the filet may be served *al limone* or with lemon wedges. The dish is typically served with a side vegetable or pasta.

Gluten-Free Decision Factors:
- Ensure no wheat flour in sauce
- Ensure no wheat flour pasta—order gluten-free pasta or polenta if available

Food Allergen Preparation Considerations:
- Food allergens may vary in side vegetables
- Contains fish from salmon
- May contain corn from vegetable oil
- May contain dairy from butter and sauce
- May contain eggs from pasta
- May contain peanuts from vegetable oil
- May contain soy from vegetable oil
- May contain tree nuts from sauce

Scampi (Prawns)

Scampi simply means prawns; extremely large ones called *mazzancolle* are very popular in Rome. In most cases, they are sautéed in butter or olive oil with white wine, garlic, salt, pepper and topped with minced basil or parsley. Cream and lemon juice are other ingredients used occasionally when prepared in this style. *Fra diavolo* (sautéed in a spicy tomato sauce) and *al forno* (baked in tomato sauce and topped with cheese) are other common variations. If baked, although uncommon, bread crumbs may be present. Scampi is often served with pasta as a side dish.

Gluten-Free Decision Factors:

- Ensure no wheat flour in sauce

- Ensure no bread crumbs

- Ensure no wheat flour pasta—order gluten-free pasta or polenta if available

Food Allergen Preparation Considerations:

- Contains shellfish from shrimp

- May contain corn from bread crumbs and vegetable oil

- May contain dairy from bread crumbs, butter, cheese, cream and sauce

- May contain eggs from bread crumbs and pasta

- May contain peanuts from bread crumbs and vegetable oil

- May contain soy from bread crumbs and vegetable oil

- May contain tree nuts from bread crumbs and sauce

Side Dishes
Broccoli Rabe (Broccoli Florets)

Broccoli Rabe is a slightly bitter tasting relative of broccoli. It is also called *brocoletti di rape, rape* and *rapini*. It resembles the leafy flower of regular broccoli and is very popular in Southern Italy. Outside of Italy, many restaurants may substitute *broccoli rabe* with regular broccoli. The Italian preference is to boil *broccoli rabe* for a few minutes to take out the bitterness, then sauté it in olive oil with garlic, salt and chili peppers. In Northern Italian restaurants, butter may be added along with various Italian herbs. The dish is usually garnished with chopped parsley and sometimes lemon wedges.

Gluten-Free Decision Factors:
- None

Food Allergen Preparation Considerations:
- May contain corn from vegetable oil
- May contain dairy from butter
- May contain peanuts from vegetable oil
- May contain soy from vegetable oil

Funghi all' Aglio e Olio (Mushrooms in Garlic and Olive Oil)

Mushrooms are a very popular Italian side dish, with this style being the most common in restaurants. Mushrooms such as cremini, porcini and portabella are sautéed in olive oil, garlic, salt and pepper. In Northern Italian restaurants, butter may be added along with various Italian herbs and bread crumbs. The dish is usually garnished with chopped parsley.

Gluten-Free Decision Factors:
- Ensure no wheat flour as ingredient
- Ensure no bread crumbs

Food Allergen Preparation Considerations:

- May contain corn from bread crumbs and vegetable oil

- May contain dairy from bread crumbs and butter

- May contain eggs from bread crumbs

- May contain peanuts from bread crumbs and vegetable oil

- May contain soy from bread crumbs and vegetable oil

- May contain tree nuts from bread crumbs

Melanzane alla Griglia (Grilled Eggplant)

Italian cuisine features eggplant more than most international cuisines, with grilled being one of the more common styles of preparation. Slices of eggplant are marinated in garlic, olive oil, salt and pepper, then scored and grilled over an open flame. In some cases, the eggplant may be dusted with wheat flour or coated with bread crumbs. Grilled eggplant is usually garnished with chopped parsley.

Gluten-Free Decision Factors:
- Ensure eggplant is not dusted with wheat flour

- Ensure no bread crumbs

Food Allergen Preparation Considerations:
- May contain corn from bread crumbs and vegetable oil

- May contain dairy from bread crumbs

- May contain eggs from bread crumbs

- May contain peanuts from bread crumbs and vegetable oil

- May contain soy from bread crumbs and vegetable oil

- May contain tree nuts from bread crumbs

Polenta (Boiled Corn Meal)

Polenta has been a starch staple in Northern Italy for hundreds of years, far more so than pasta. The standard preparation involves boiling corn meal in water with salt. Once the water has been boiled out, the corn meal is malleable and can be formed into many different shapes. Depending on the restaurant, you may see *polenta* served on the side topped with butter and various Italian cheeses. It may also be cut into sticks or wedges and fried crisp in oil. Grilling is another popular preparation style. *Polenta* also serves as an excellent substitute for pasta when available and can be topped with any type of standard Italian sauce.

Gluten-Free Decision Factors:
- Ensure no wheat flour in sauce
- Ensure oil used for frying is designated for polenta only and is not used to fry other items that may be battered or dusted with wheat flour

Food Allergen Preparation Considerations:
- Contains corn from corn meal and possibly from vegetable oil
- May contain dairy from butter, cheese and sauce
- May contain peanuts from vegetable oil
- May contain soy from vegetable oil
- May contain tree nuts from sauce

Desserts
Frutti di Stagione (Fresh Fruit in Season)

Italians love fresh fruit and generally only eat fruit when it is in season. Apples, berries, melons and oranges are usually available, but any combination of fruit can be offered. The fruit may be served plain or topped with whipped cream or *zabaglione*, an Italian custard.

Gluten-Free Decision Factors:
  • None

Food Allergen Preparation Considerations:
  • May contain dairy from whipped cream

  • May contain eggs from custard

Gelato (Italian Ice Cream or Sherbet)

Gelato is somewhere between ice cream and sherbet. There are many flavors including chocolate, custard, fruits and nuts. Many restaurants make it fresh in their kitchens, while others may opt to purchase pre-fabricated *gelato*. Puréed fruit or other natural flavors and sugar are mixed with heavy whipping cream and frozen, either in a freezer or in an ice cream machine. As is the case with most ice cream, ask your server to read the ingredients listed on the container if available and keep your flavor choices simple. Gelato may be served with a cookie.

Gluten-Free Decision Factors:

- Ensure no stabilizers which may contain gluten

- Request no cookie

Food Allergen Preparation Considerations:

- Contains dairy as an ingredient and possibly from cookie

- May contain corn from colors or flavors

- May contain eggs from cookie and colors or flavors

- May contain peanuts from cookie and various flavors

- May contain soy from cookie and colors or flavors

- May contain tree nuts from cookie and various flavors

Granita (Italian Ice)

It was known as *Ghiaccio Italiano* (Italian ice) in the immigrant neighborhoods of New York City, as well as in other cities on the east coast of the US for the first half of the 20th century. *Granita* is still found on the streets of Italy, as well as in restaurants. It is shaved ice with fruit syrup poured over the top, rather like a snow cone. What separates it from the standard snow cone in Italy is that the syrups are made fresh. Fruit is puréed and boiled with sugar and sometimes wine or liquor added to flavor the syrup.

Gluten-Free Decision Factors:
- Ensure no malt or stabilizers which may contain gluten

Food Allergen Preparation Considerations:
- May contain corn from colors or flavors
- May contain soy from colors or flavors

Zabaglione (Italian Custard)

Unlike most custards, *zabaglione* is usually free of dairy products. It is made by whipping egg yolks and sugar together while cooking in a double boiler. Sweet *Marsala* wine is added toward the end of this process. When finished, it resembles a thick whipped cream with a yellow tint. *Zabaglione* is served warm or chilled, by itself or over fresh fruit. It may also be served on top of cake.

Gluten-Free Decision Factors:
- Ensure no cake

Food Allergen Preparation Considerations:
- Contains eggs from egg yolks and possibly from cake

- May contain dairy from cake

- May contain peanuts from cake

- May contain tree nuts from cake

Italian Cuisine:
Quick Reference Guide
(Appetizers – Soups)

	Corn	Dairy	Eggs	Fish	Gluten/Wheat	Peanuts	Shellfish	Soy	Tree Nuts
Appetizers									
Calamari alla Griglia (Grilled Calamari)	O	O	O		O	O	●	O	O
Carpaccio di Manzo (Beef Carpaccio)	O	●			O		O		
Carpaccio di Salmone (Salmon Carpaccio)	O			●	O	O		O	
Cocktail di Gamberi (Shrimp Cocktail)	O		O	O	O		●	O	
Cozze al Vapore (Steamed Mussels)	O	●	O	O	O	O	O	●	O	O
Prosciutto e Melone (Cured Ham and Melon)		O							
Soups									
Gazpaccio	O		O		O				

Always ensure no cross-contamination in food preparation

● Typically contains allergen   O May contain allergen

Italian Cuisine:
Quick Reference Guide
(Salads – Italian Specialties)

	Corn	Dairy	Eggs	Fish	Gluten/Wheat	Peanuts	Shellfish	Soy	Tree Nuts
Salads									
Insalata Caprese (Mozzarella Tomato Salad)	O	●				O		O	
Insalata Mista (Mixed Green Salad)	O		O	O	O	O		O	
Italian Specialties									
Risotto ai Frutti di Mare (Arborio Rice and Seafood Dish)	O	●		●	O	O	●	O	
Risotto ai Funghi (Arborio Rice and Mushroom Dish)	O	●			O	O		O	
Risotto al Pollo (Arborio Rice and Chicken Dish)	O	●			O	O		O	
Risotto ai Quattro Formaggi (Arborio Rice and Cheese Dish)	O	●			O	O		O	

Always ensure no cross-contamination in food preparation

● Typically contains allergen   O May contain allergen

Italian Cuisine:
Quick Reference Guide
(Meat Entrees – Chicken Entrees)

	Corn	Dairy	Eggs	Fish	Gluten/Wheat	Peanuts	Shellfish	Soy	Tree Nuts
Meat Entrees									
Costatella D'Agnello (Rack of Lamb)*	O	O	O		O	O		O	O
Fileto di Manzo (Filet Mignon)*	O	O	O		O	O		O	
Medalione di Manzo (Beef Tenderloin Medallions)*	O	O	O		O	O		O	O
Vitello (Veal)*	O	O	O		O	O		O	O
Chicken Entrees									
Petti di Pollo (Chicken Breast)*	O	O	O		O	O		O	O
Pollo Arrosto Rosmarino (Rosemary Roasted Chicken)*	O	O	O		O	O		O	O

Always ensure no cross-contamination in food preparation

● Typically contains allergen   O May contain allergen

* Food allergens may vary depending upon type of accompaniment

Italian Cuisine:
Quick Reference Guide
(Seafood Entrees – Side Dishes)

	Corn	Dairy	Eggs	Fish	Gluten/Wheat	Peanuts	Shellfish	Soy	Tree Nuts
Seafood Entrees									
Salmone alla Griglia (Grilled Salmon)*	O	O	O	●	O	O		O	O
Scampi (Prawns)	O	O	O		O	O	●	O	O
Side Dishes									
Broccoli Rabe (Broccoli Florets)	O	O				O		O	
Funghi all' Aglio e Olio (Mushrooms in Garlic and Olive Oil)	O	O	O		O	O		O	O
Melanzane alla Griglia (Grilled Eggplant)	O	O	O		O	O		O	O
Polenta (Boiled Corn Meal)	●	O			O	O		O	O

Always ensure no cross-contamination in food preparation

●   Typically contains allergen   O   May contain allergen

*   Food allergens may vary depending upon type of accompaniment

Italian Cuisine:
Quick Reference Guide
(Desserts)

Desserts	Corn	Dairy	Eggs	Fish	Gluten/Wheat	Peanuts	Shellfish	Soy	Tree Nuts
Frutti di Stagione (Fresh Fruit in Season)		O	O						
Gelato (Italian Ice Cream or Sherbert)	O	●	O		O	O		O	O
Granita (Italian Ice)	O				O			O	
Zabaglione (Italian Custard)		O	●		O	O		O	O

Always ensure no cross-contamination in food preparation

● Typically contains allergen   O May contain allergen

About the Authors and Additional Products

The following information highlights:

- Background of authors
- Additional books and passports

Background of Authors

Kim Koeller has spent the last 23 years eating 80% of her meals in restaurants across the globe while managing over a dozen food-related allergies/sensitivities and celiac/coeliac disease. Robert La France has spent over twelve years in the restaurant industry and devotes his spare time to a passion for the culinary arts. Collectively, they have traveled over 2 million miles across the globe, dined in 30-plus countries on four continents, and have conversational skills in French, German, Italian, Portuguese and Spanish.

Kim and Robert now promote awareness of food allergies and celiac/coeliac disease as President and Executive Vice President respectively of AllergyFree Passport™. The mission of AllergyFree Passport™, and its affiliate GlutenFree Passport™, is to empower individuals with food allergies and specialized diets to safely eat outside the home, travel and explore the world.

Be sure to view our websites for announcements of our new media products. If you would like to be included in our mailing list, obtain information on our consulting and educational services or have feedback, please contact us at:

27 North Wacker Drive, Suite 258
Chicago, IL 60606-2800
Telephone: 1- 312-952-4900
Fax: 1-312-372-2770
info@allergyfreepassport.com
http://www.allergyfreepassport.com
http://www.glutenfreepassport.com

Additional Books and Passports

As part of the *Let's Eat Out!* series, R & R Publishing has also produced a 496 page full color book —*Let's Eat Out! Your Passport to Living Gluten and Allergy Free* and other pocket-size passports designed to be carried with you anywhere and anytime. These passports include:

- American Steak & Seafood and Mexican Cuisine

- Chinese, Indian and Thai Cuisine

- Multi-Lingual Phrases

To obtain these products or to inquire about special printings, volume discount pricing and foreign rights, please contact us at:

R & R Publishing, LLC.
446 N. Wells Street, Suite 254
Chicago, IL 60610
United States
Phone: 1-312-371-4442
Toll-Free: 1-866-564-1440
Facsimile: 1-312-276-8001
info@rnrpublishing.com
http://www.rnrpublishing.com